Second Edition 2017

ISBN 9780993355042

The moral right of the author has been asserted.

All rights reserved. No part of this publication may be reproduced in any form or by any means – graphic, electronic, or mechanical including photocopying, recording taping or information storage and retrieval systems – without written permission of the copyright owner.

This book is sold subject to the condition that it shall not, by way of trade or otherwise, be lent, resold, hired out or otherwise circulated without the publisher's prior consent in any form of binding or cover other than that in which it is published and without a similar condition including this condition being imposed on the subsequent purchaser.

Copyright © 2015 by Christine Anderson

Registered With UK Copyright Service in 2015
No 284695148.

Printed by CreateSpace, An Amazon.com Company

Available from Amazon.com and other book stores

Available on Kindle and online stores

A CIP catalogue record for this book is available from the British Library.

Disclaimer

Consult your physician or other health care professional before engaging in this sugar free plan to determine if it is right for your needs. You should not subscribe to the "Sugar No More Lookbook" service if you have any type of health condition, including without limitations insulin dependent diabetes, eating disorders, cardiac insufficiency, renal insufficiency or any other concerns.

Do not start this plan if your physician or provider advises against it.

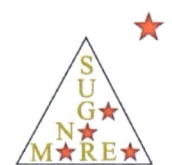

DEDICATION

This book is dedicated to all those who helped me flourish in writing.

v

SUGAR NO MORE

Christine Anderson

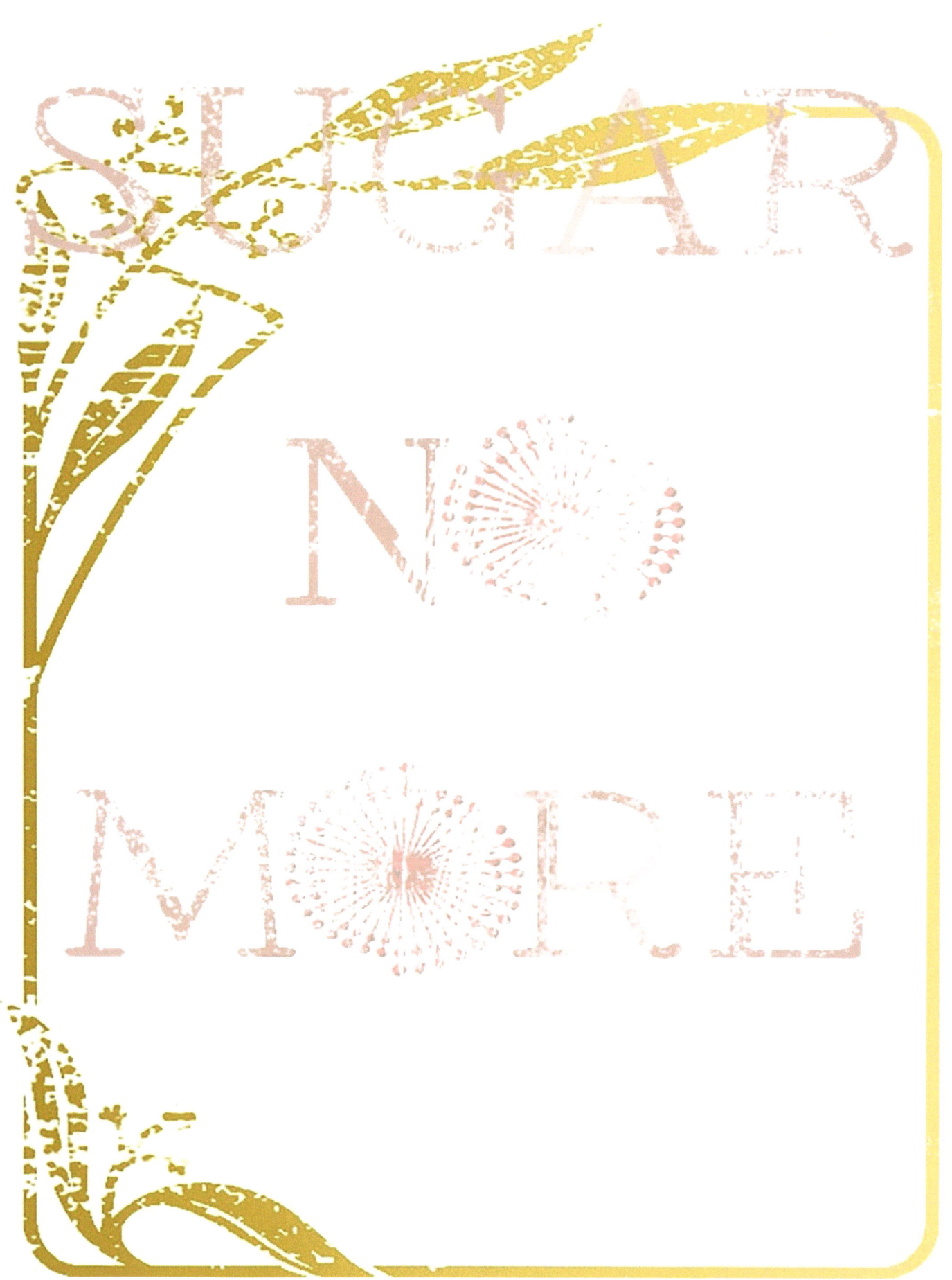

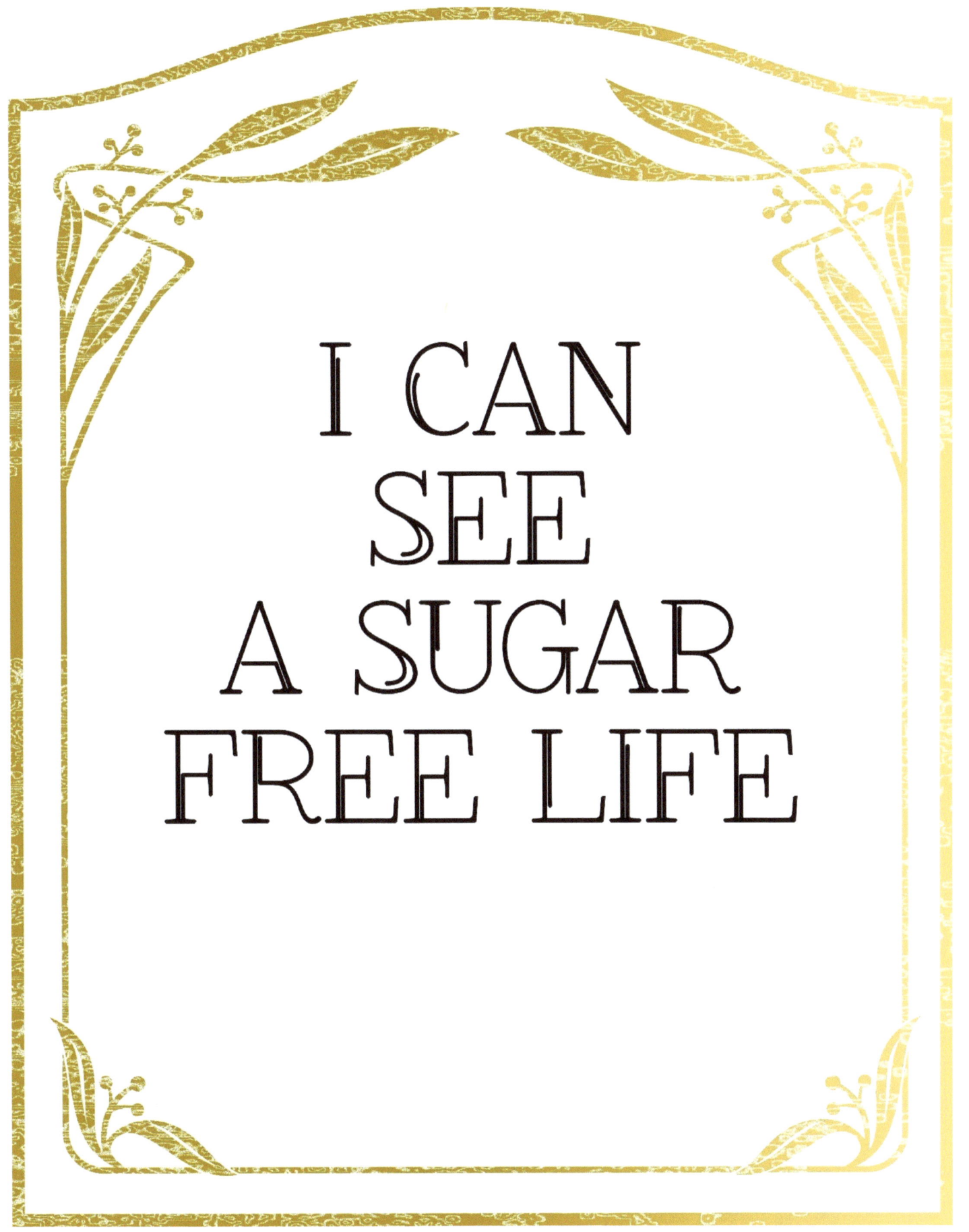

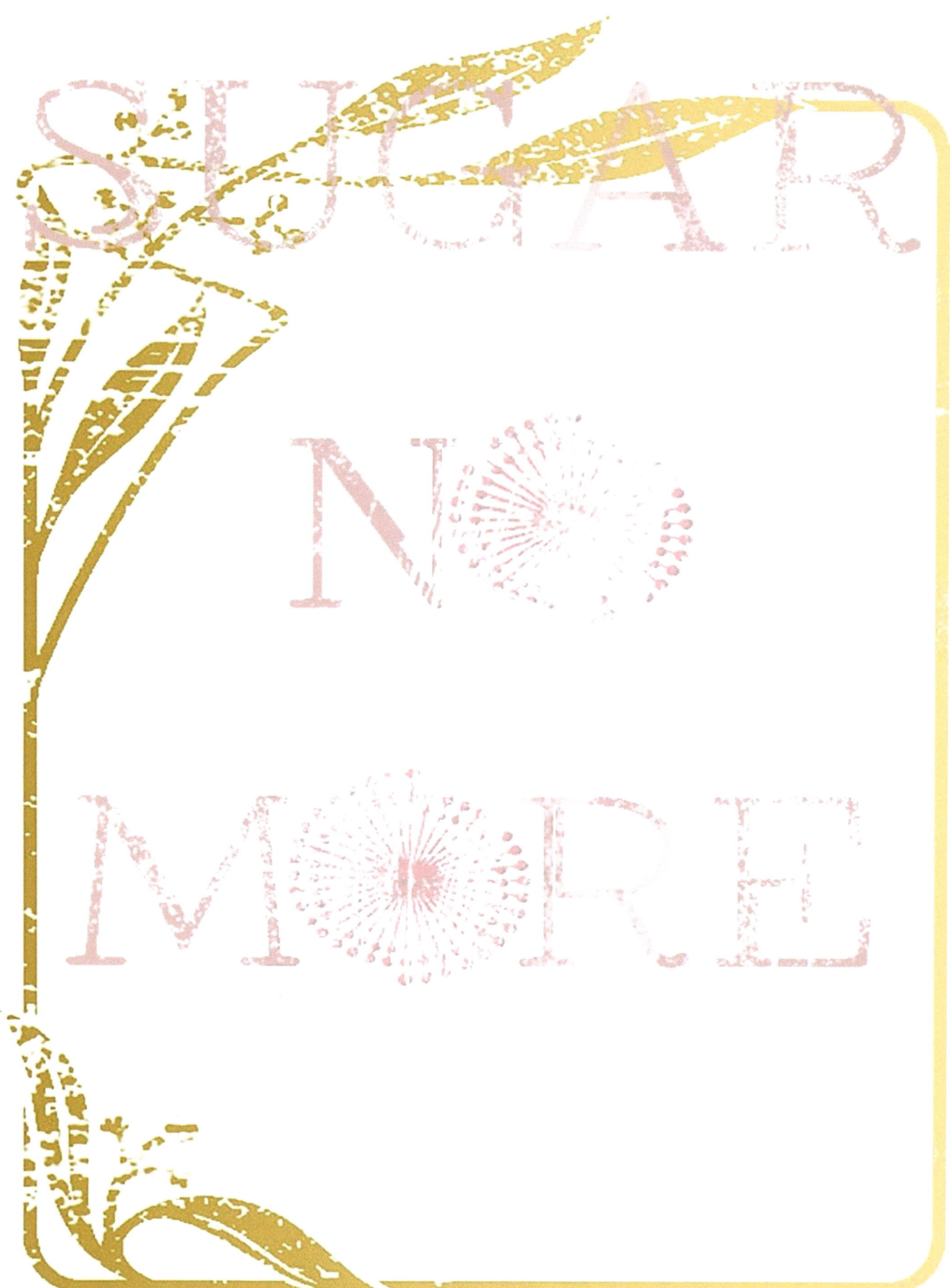

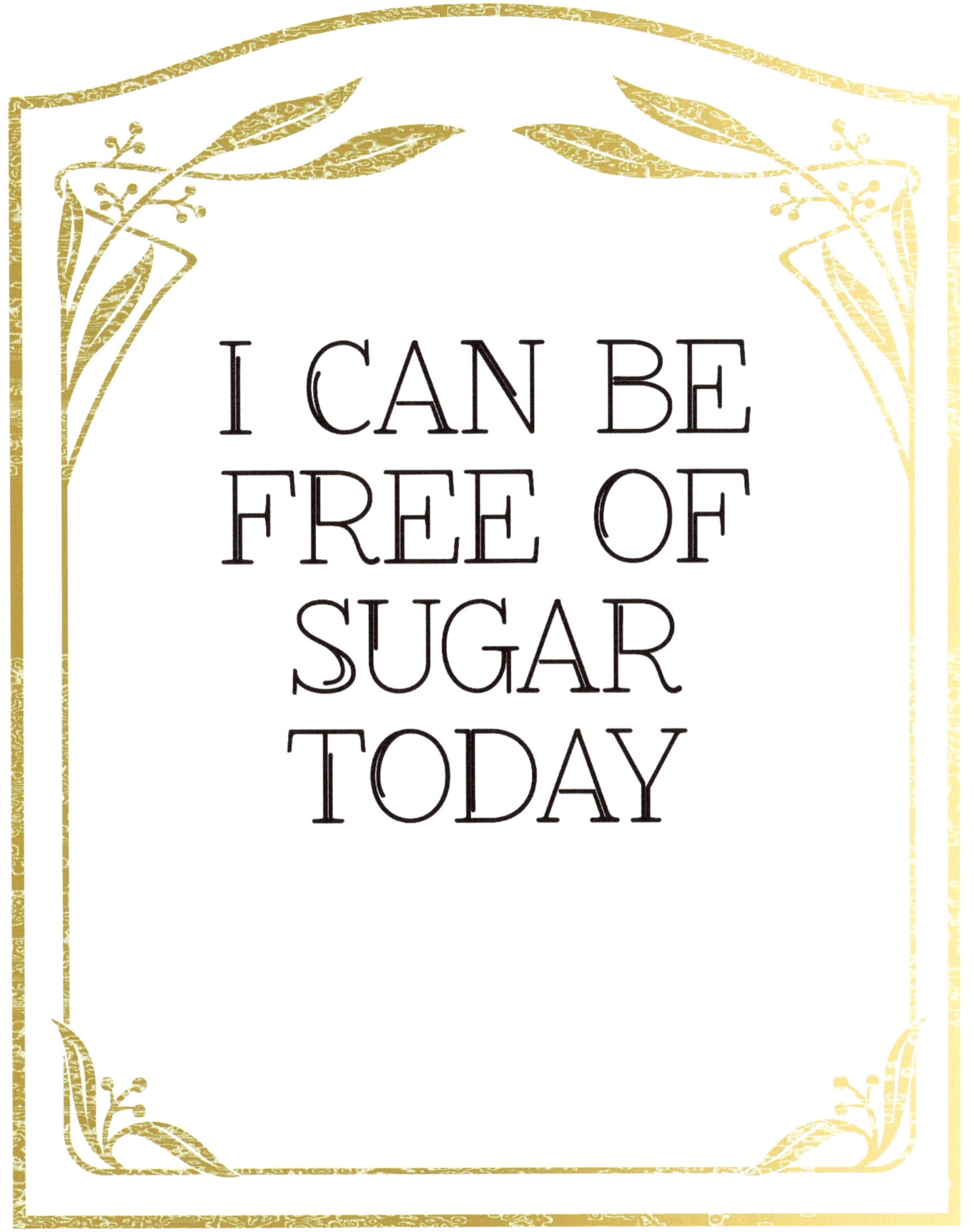

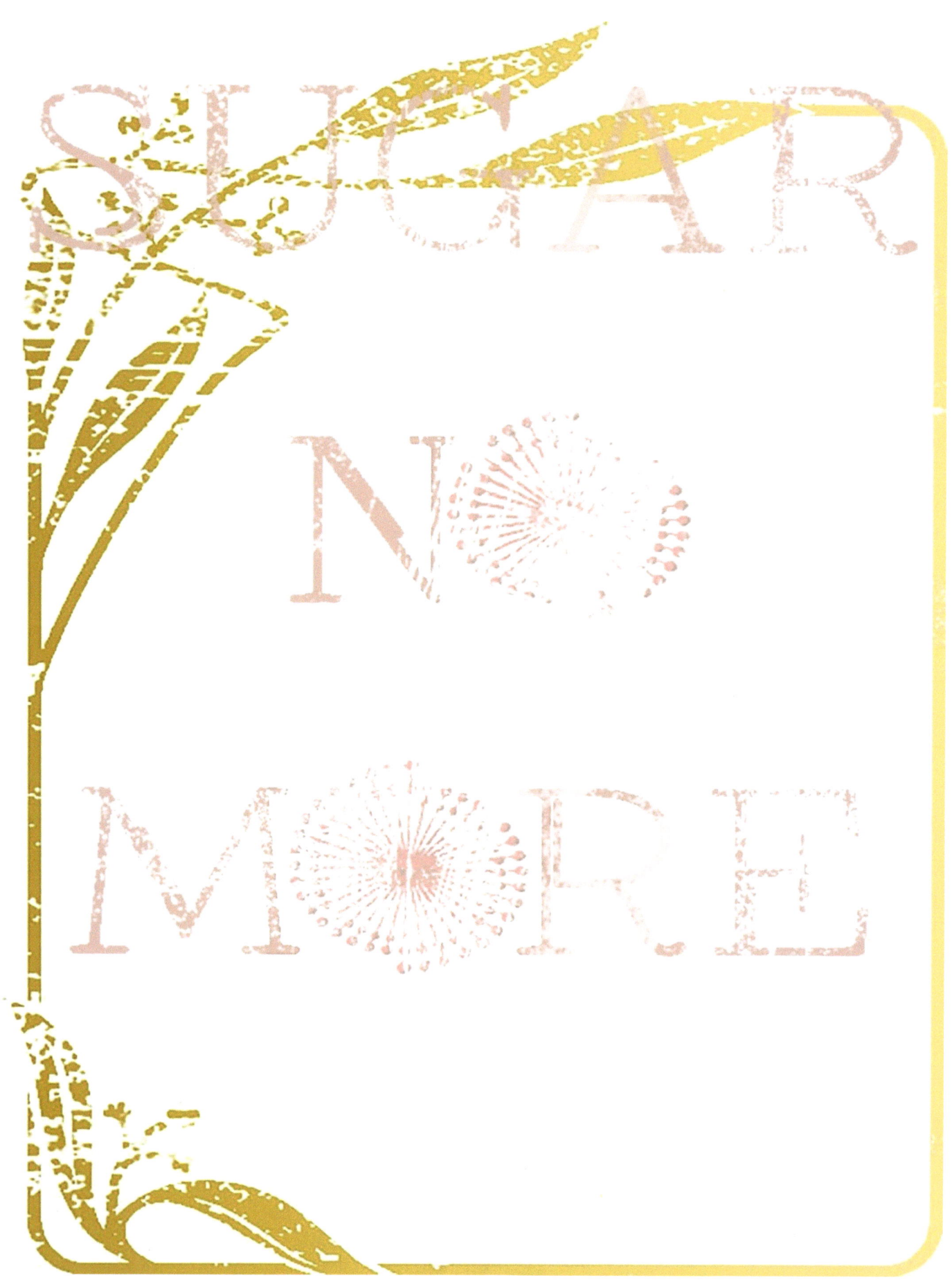

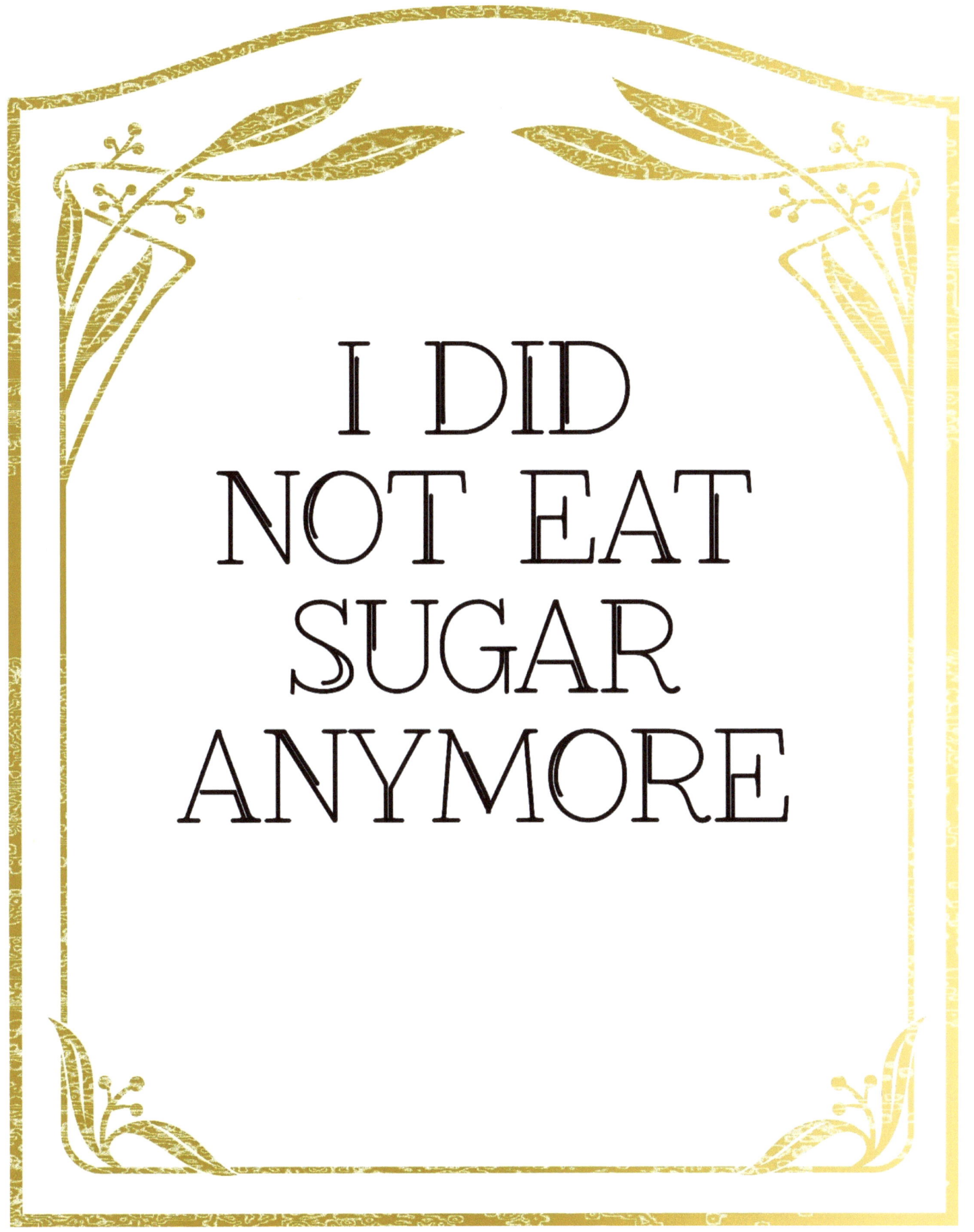

I DID NOT EAT SUGAR ANYMORE

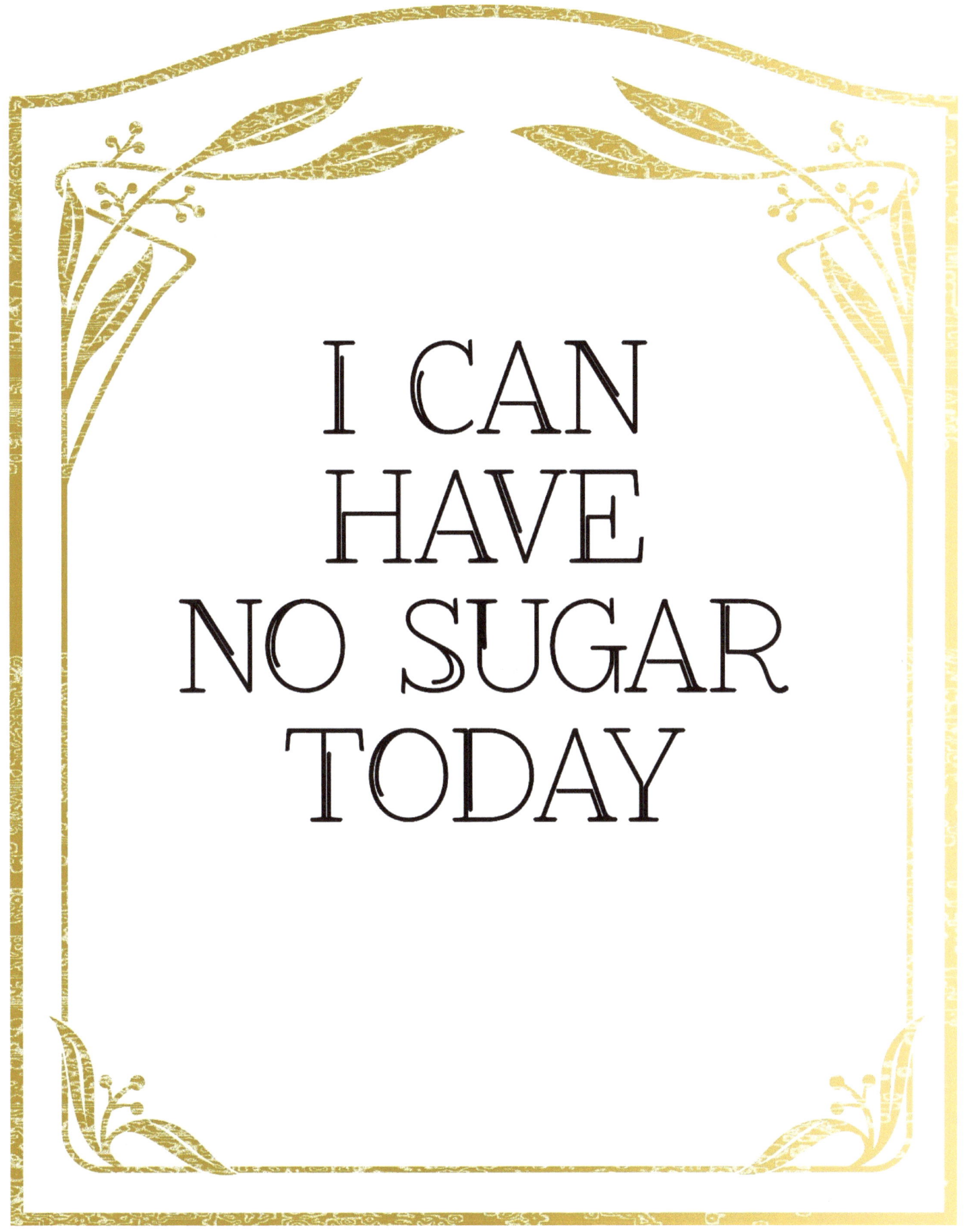

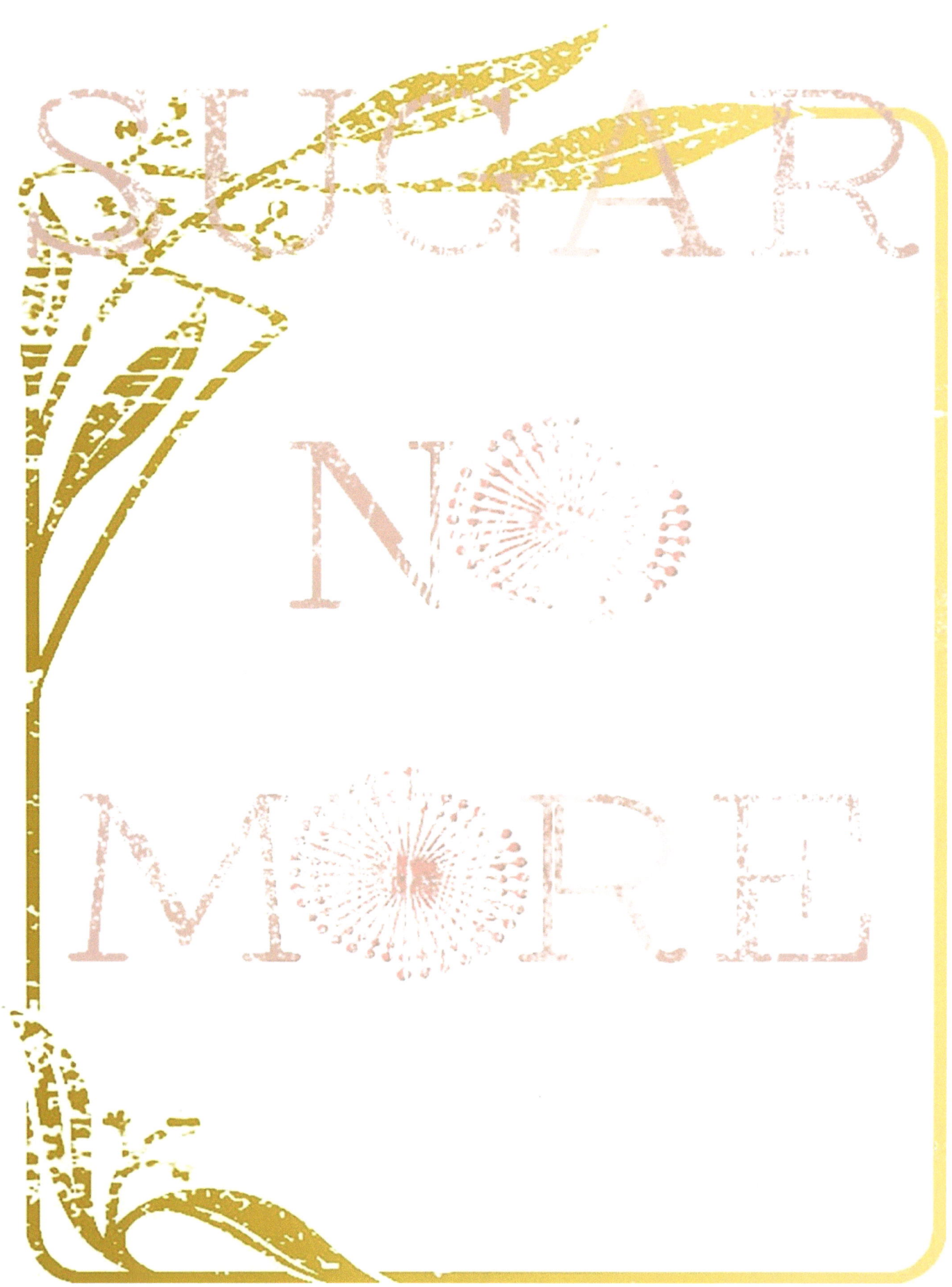

I DO NOT NEED SUGAR

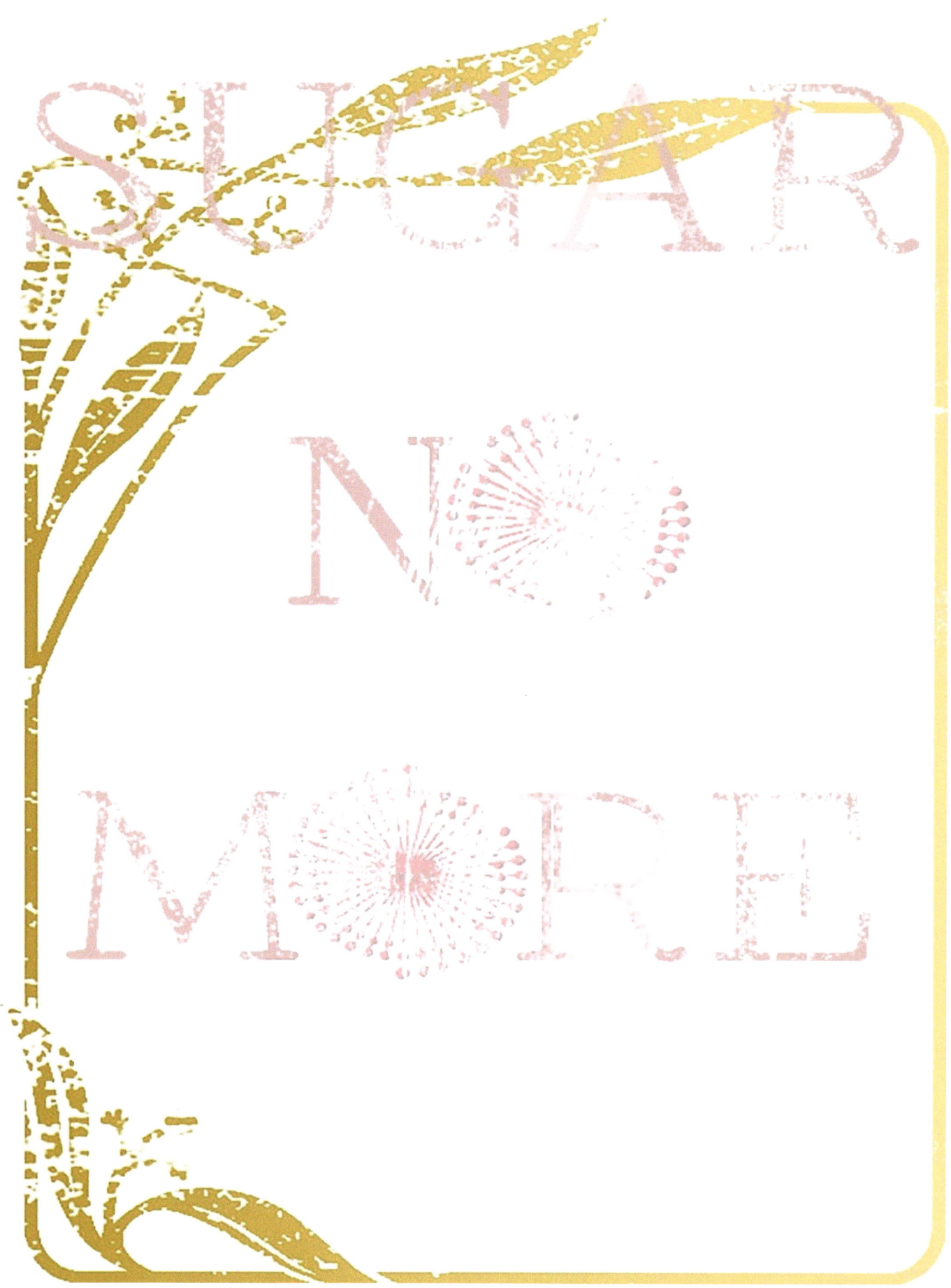

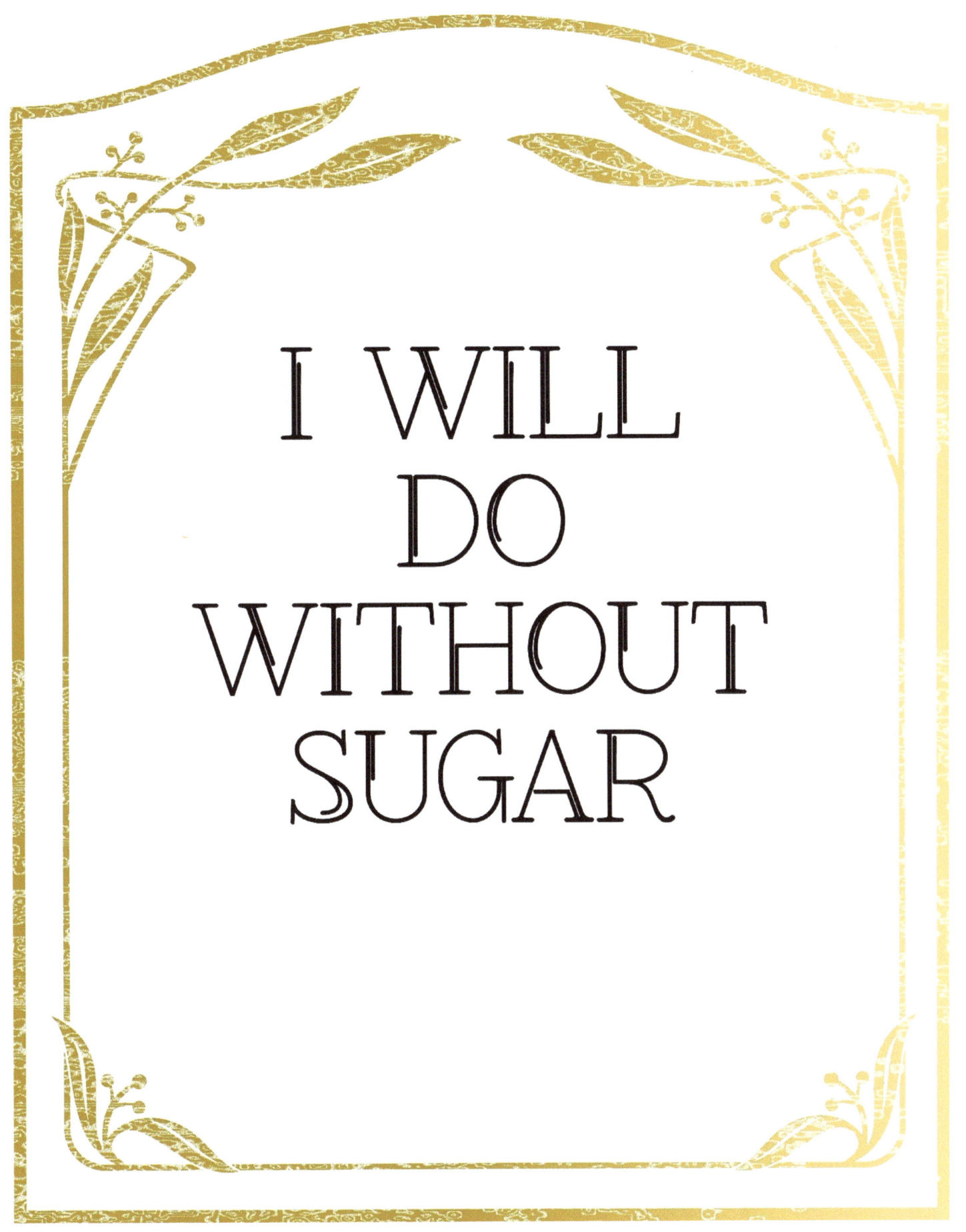

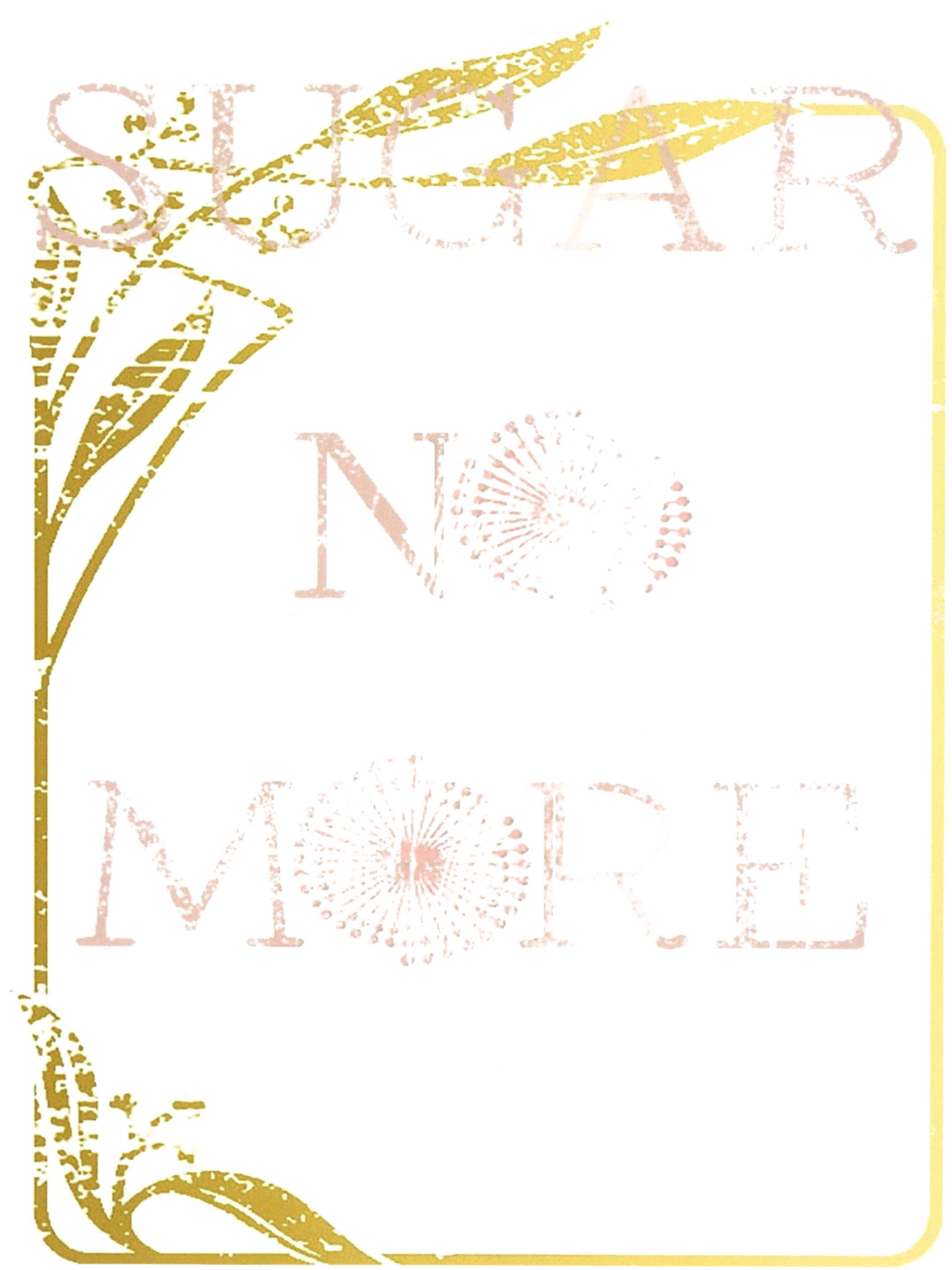

I DO NOT WANT SUGAR THE FEELING HAD GONE

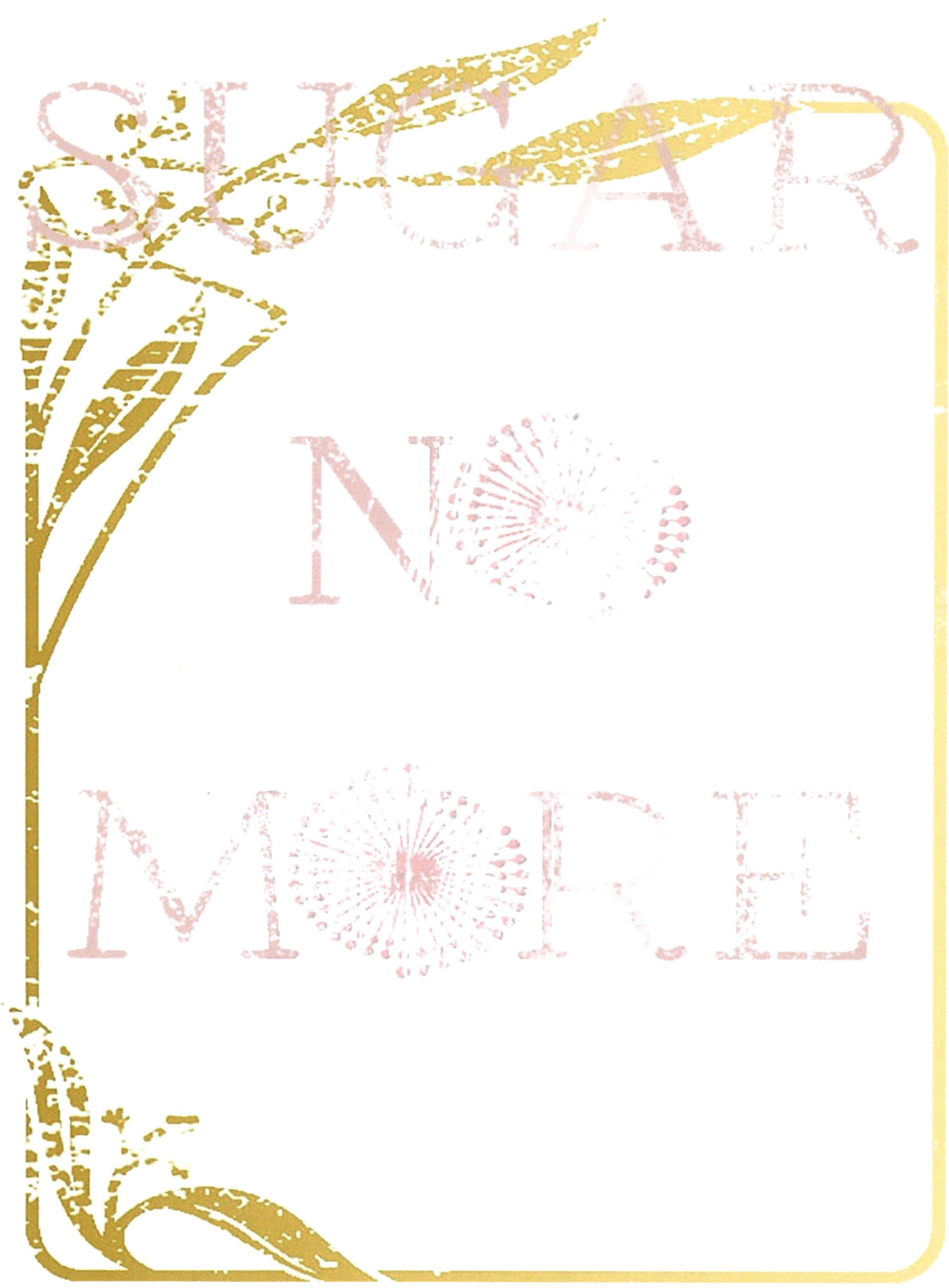

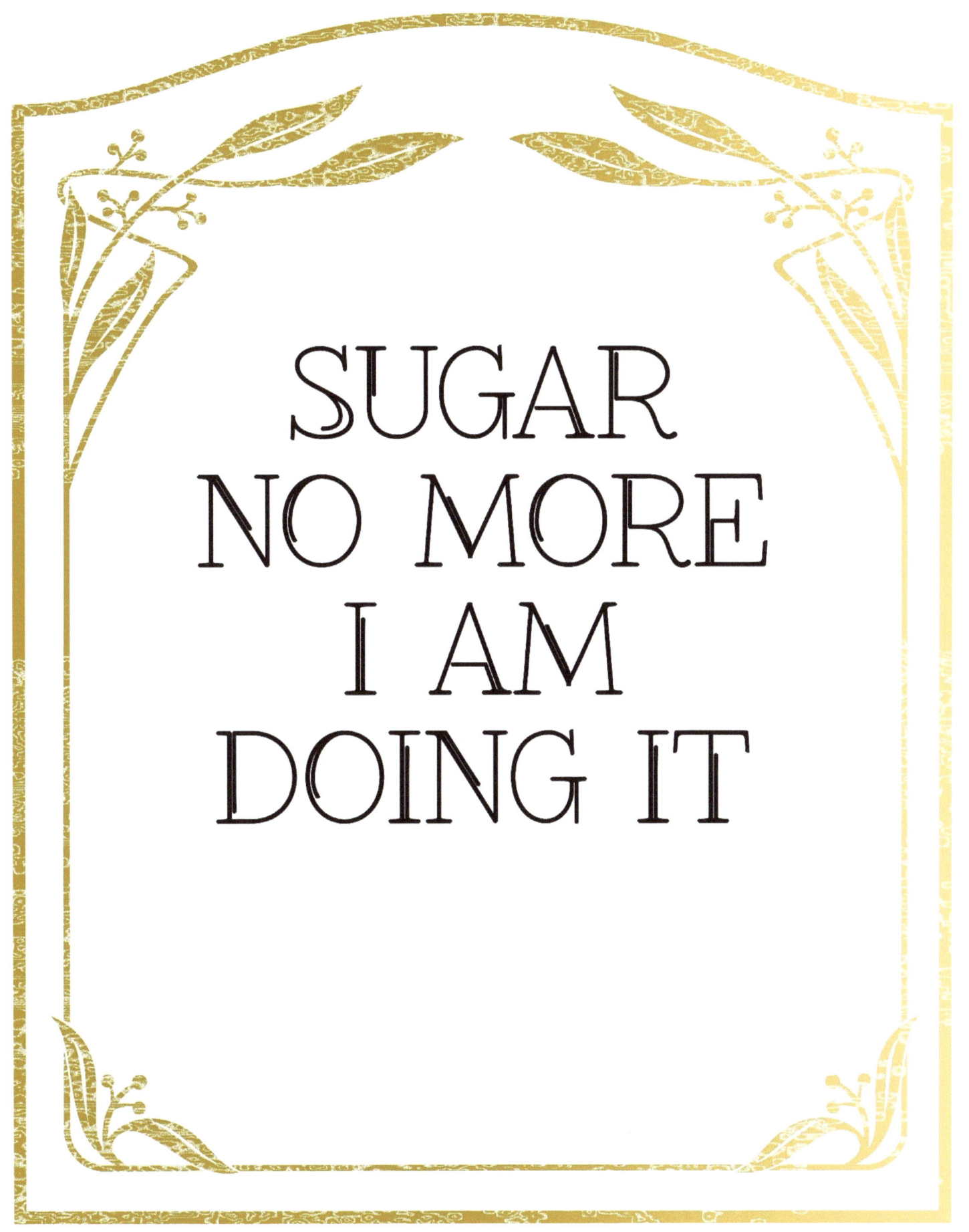

SUGAR NO MORE I AM DOING IT

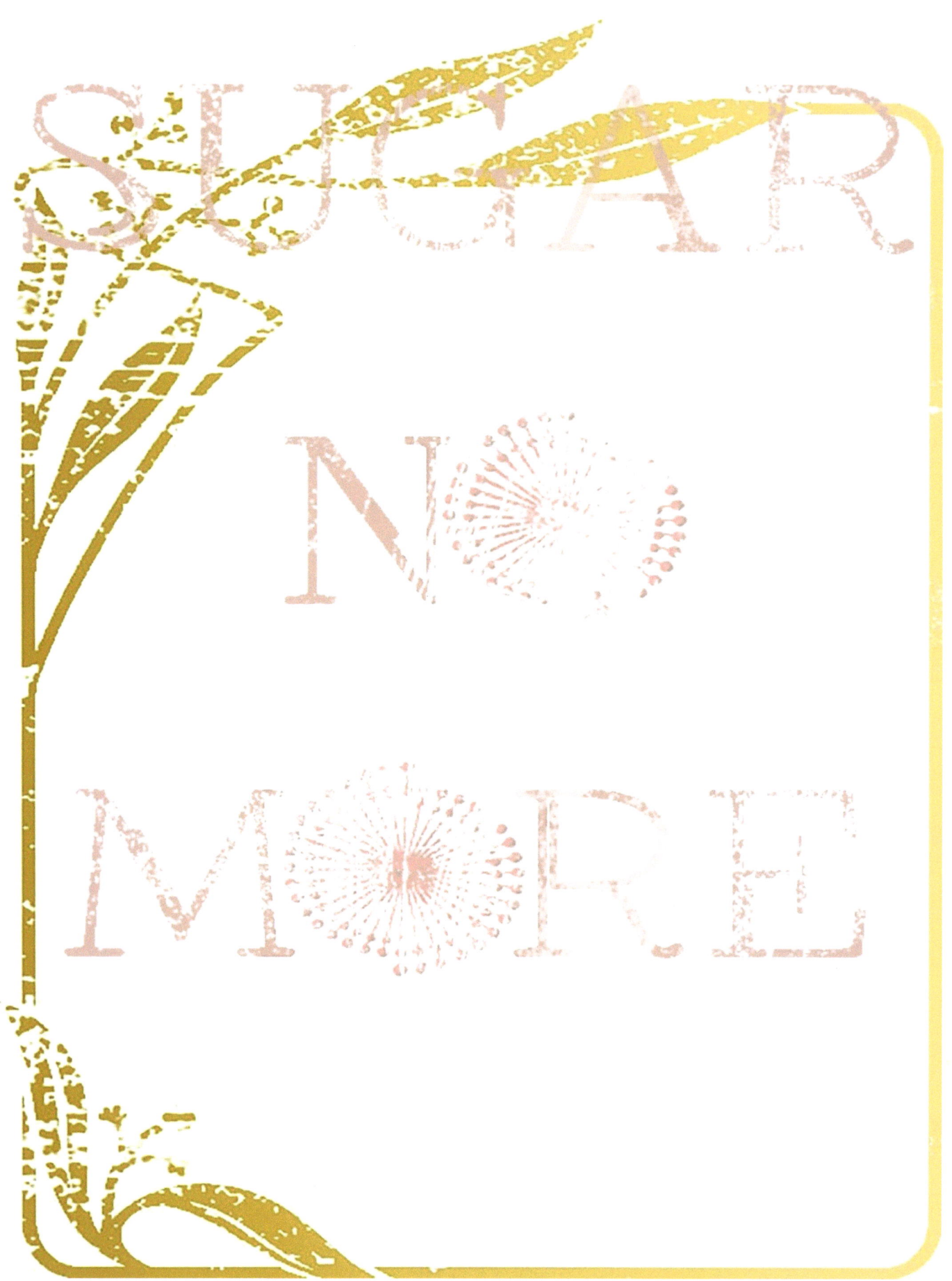

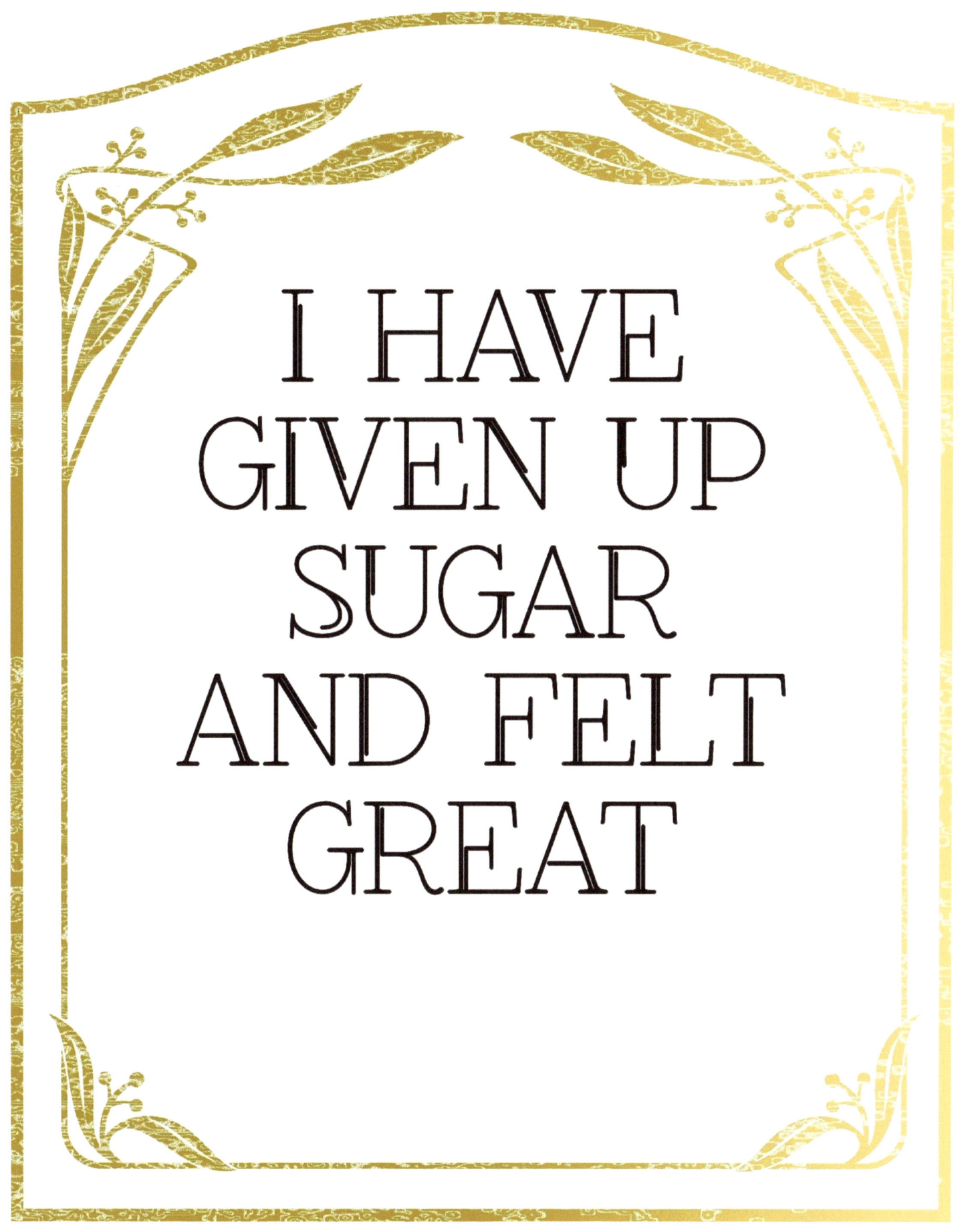

I HAVE GIVEN UP SUGAR AND FELT GREAT

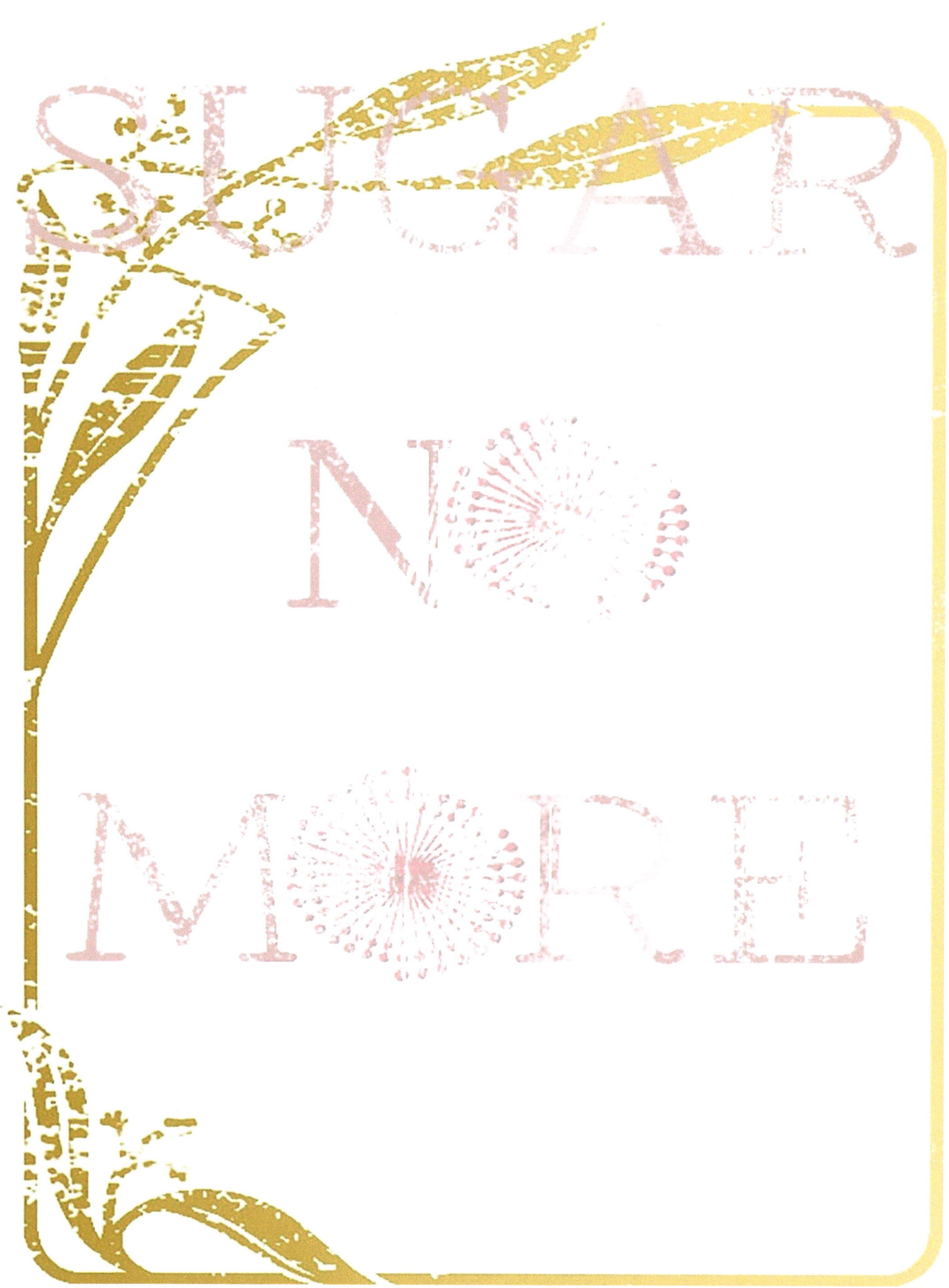

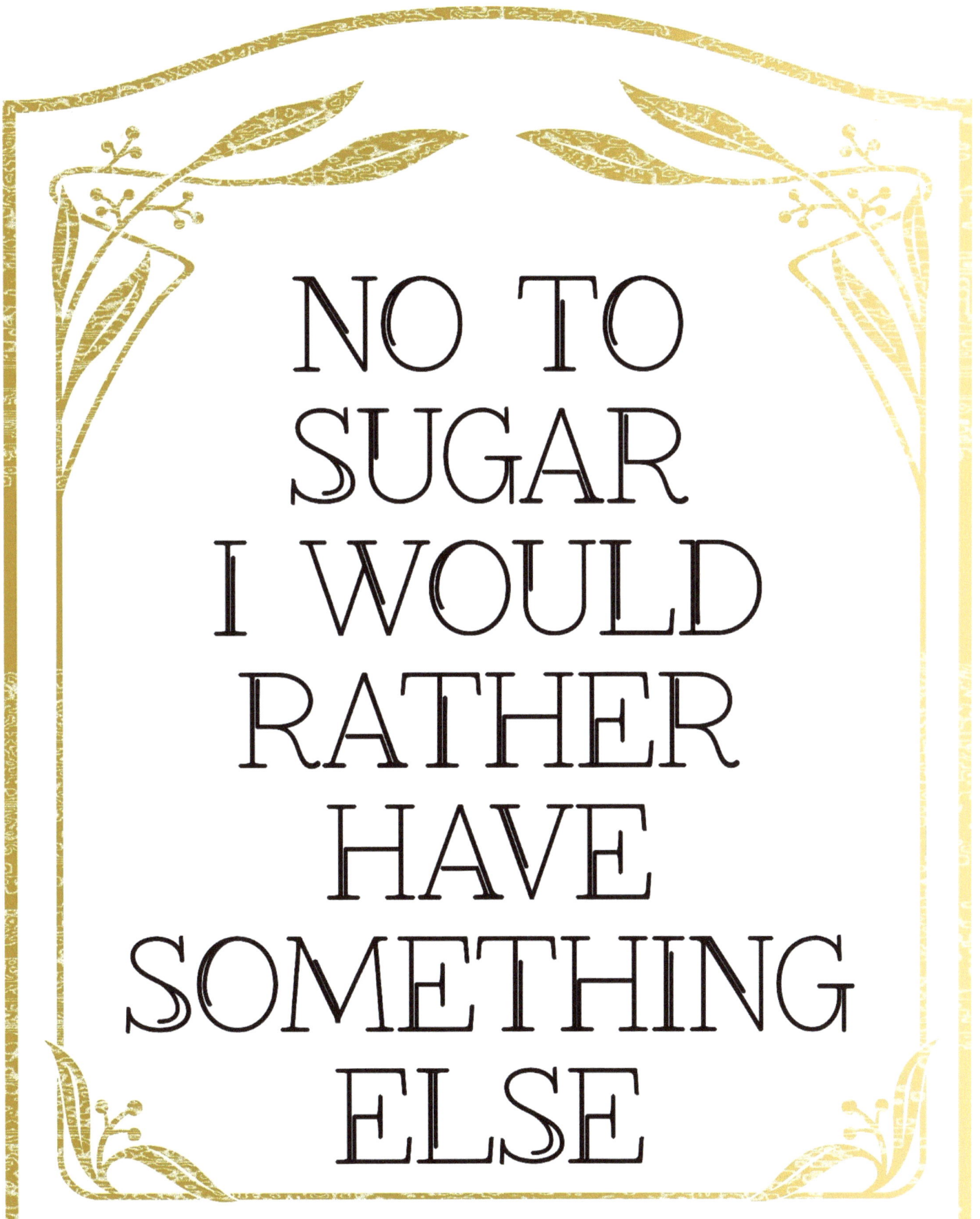

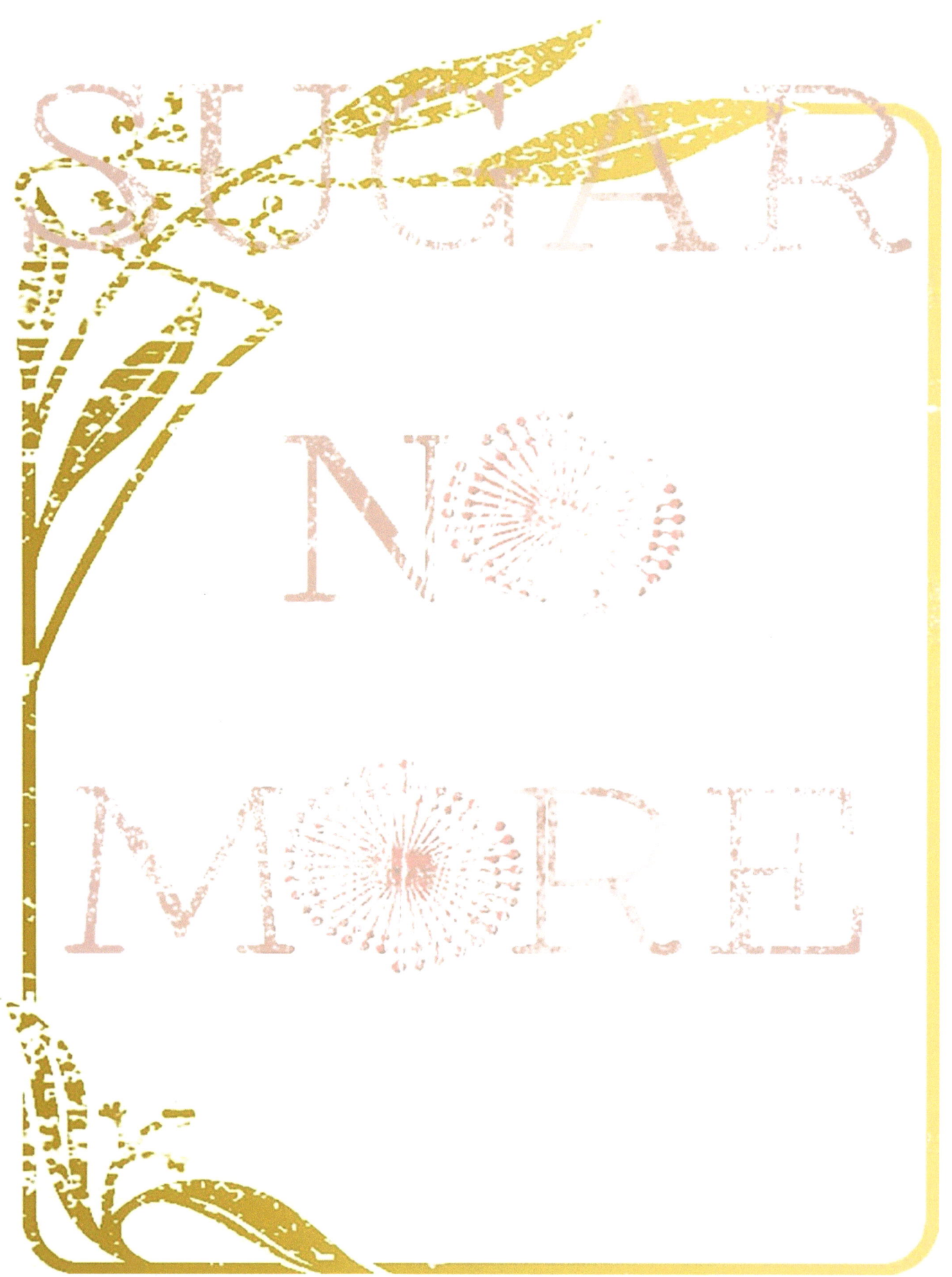

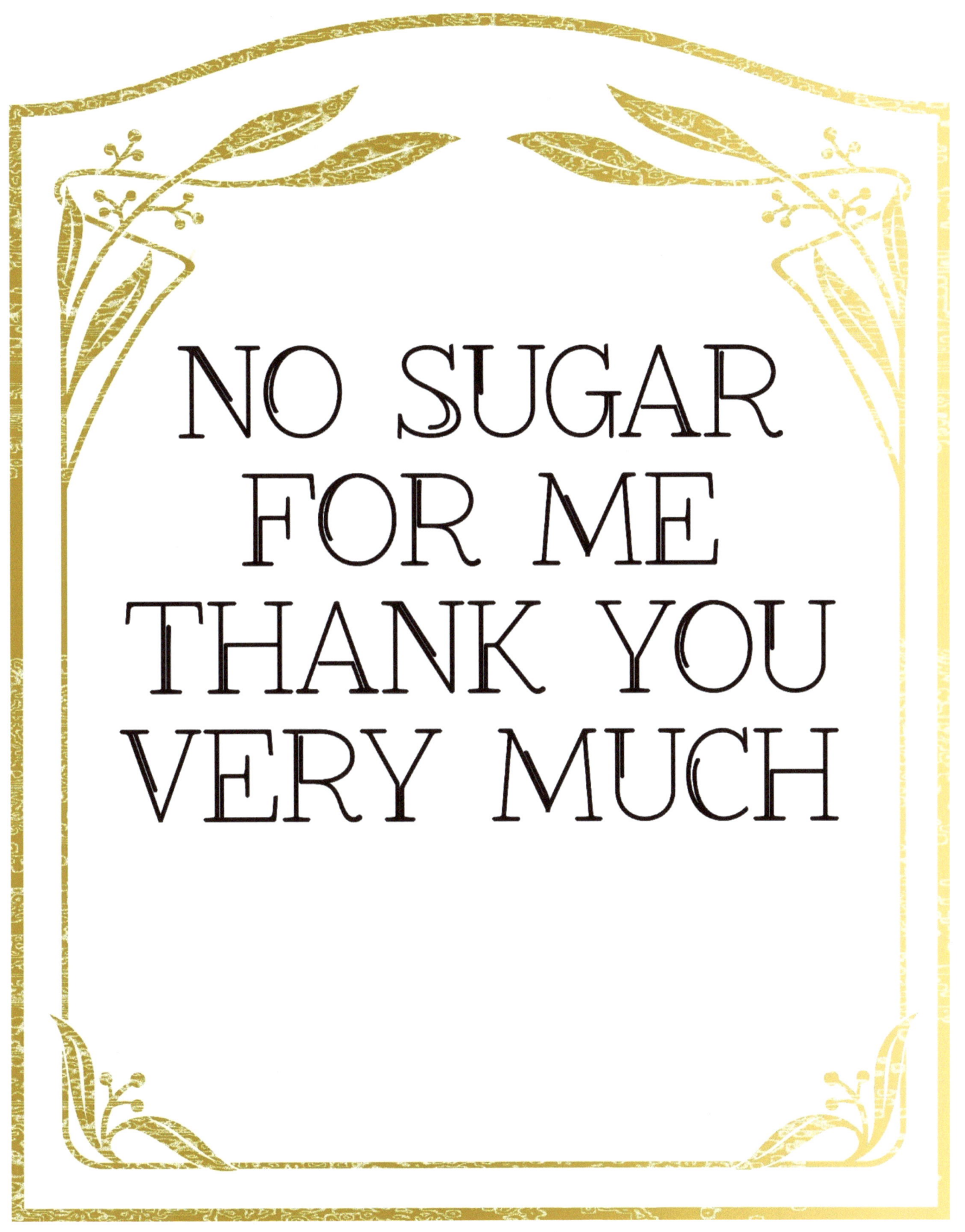

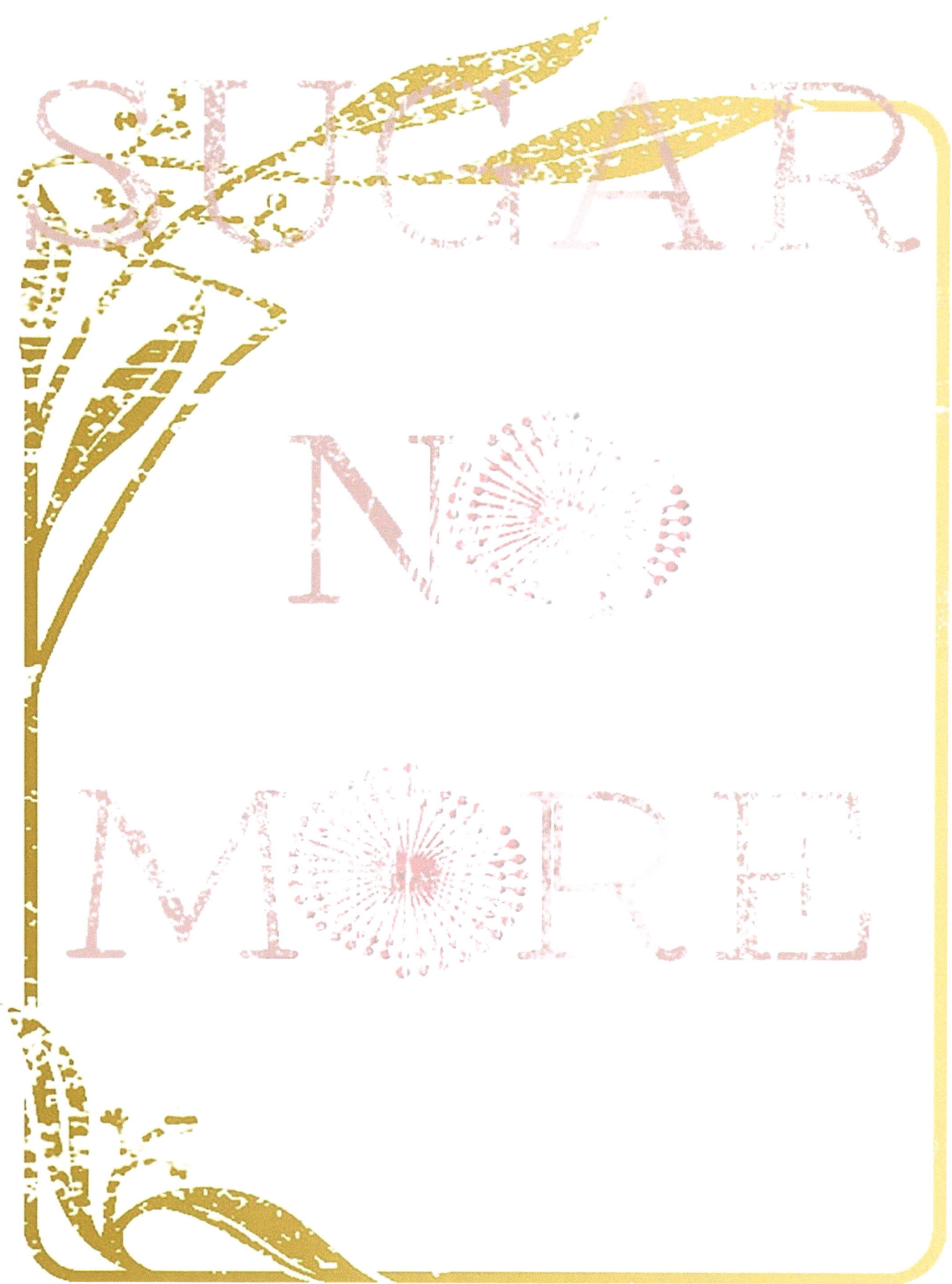

I NOW REFUSE SUGAR

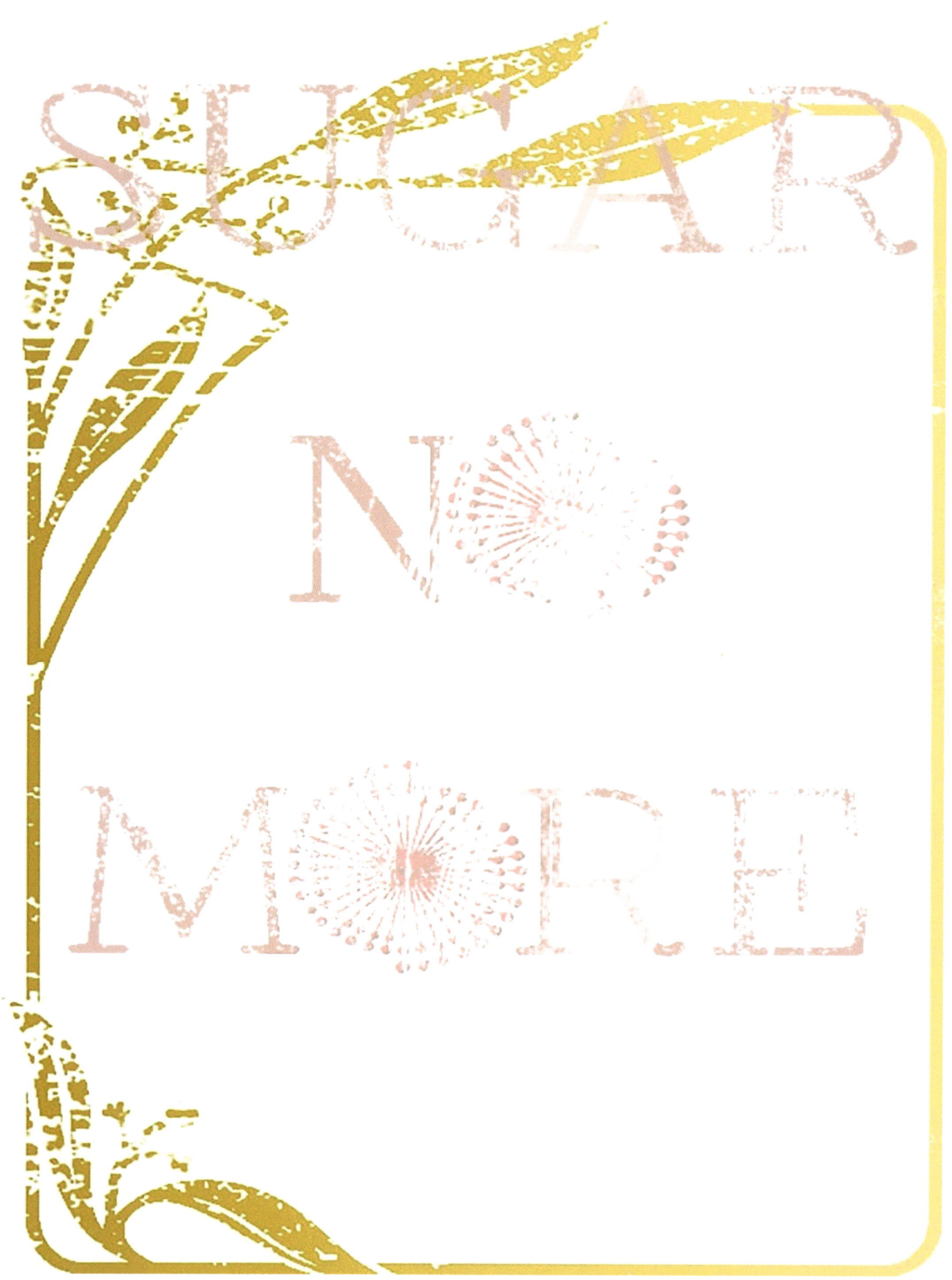

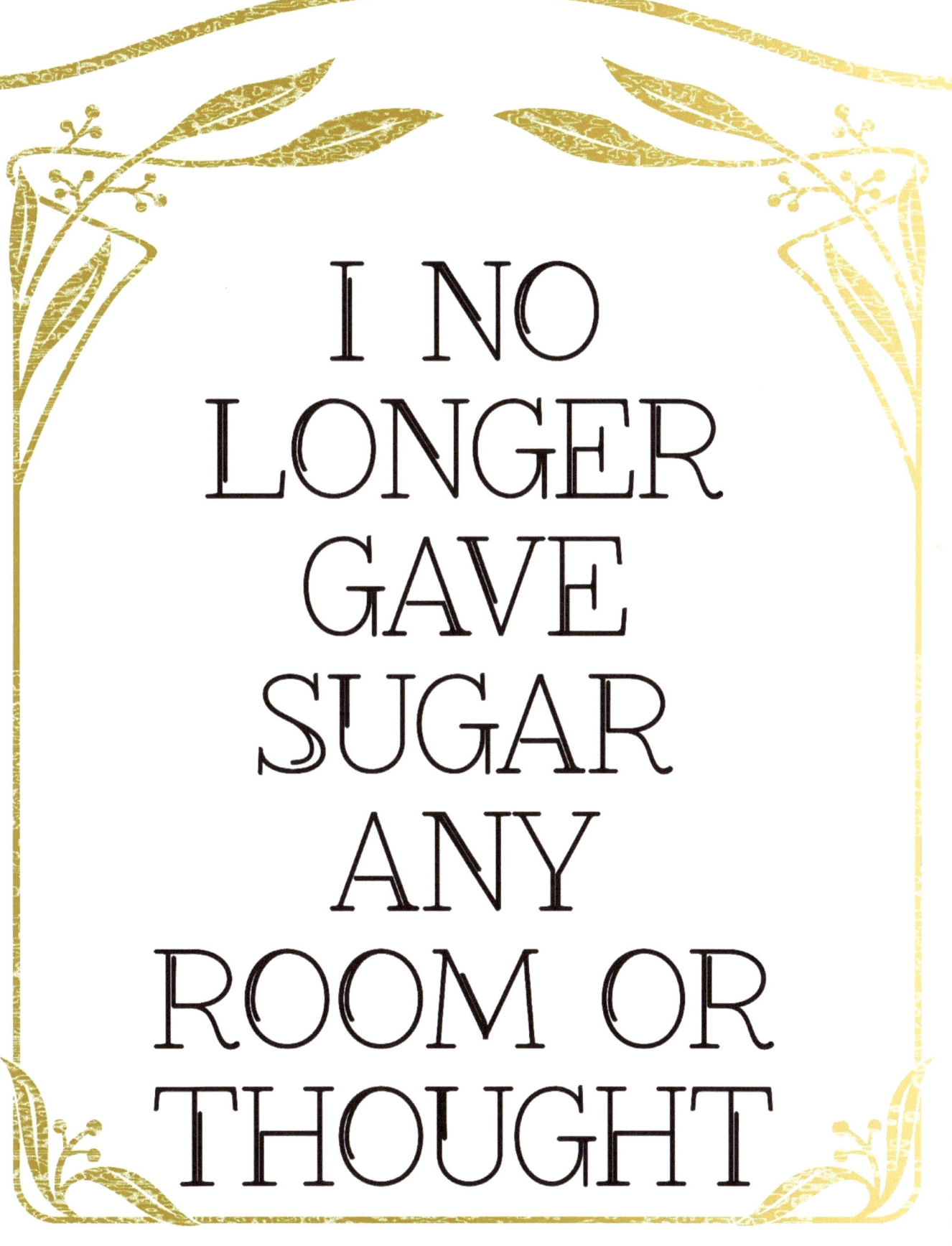

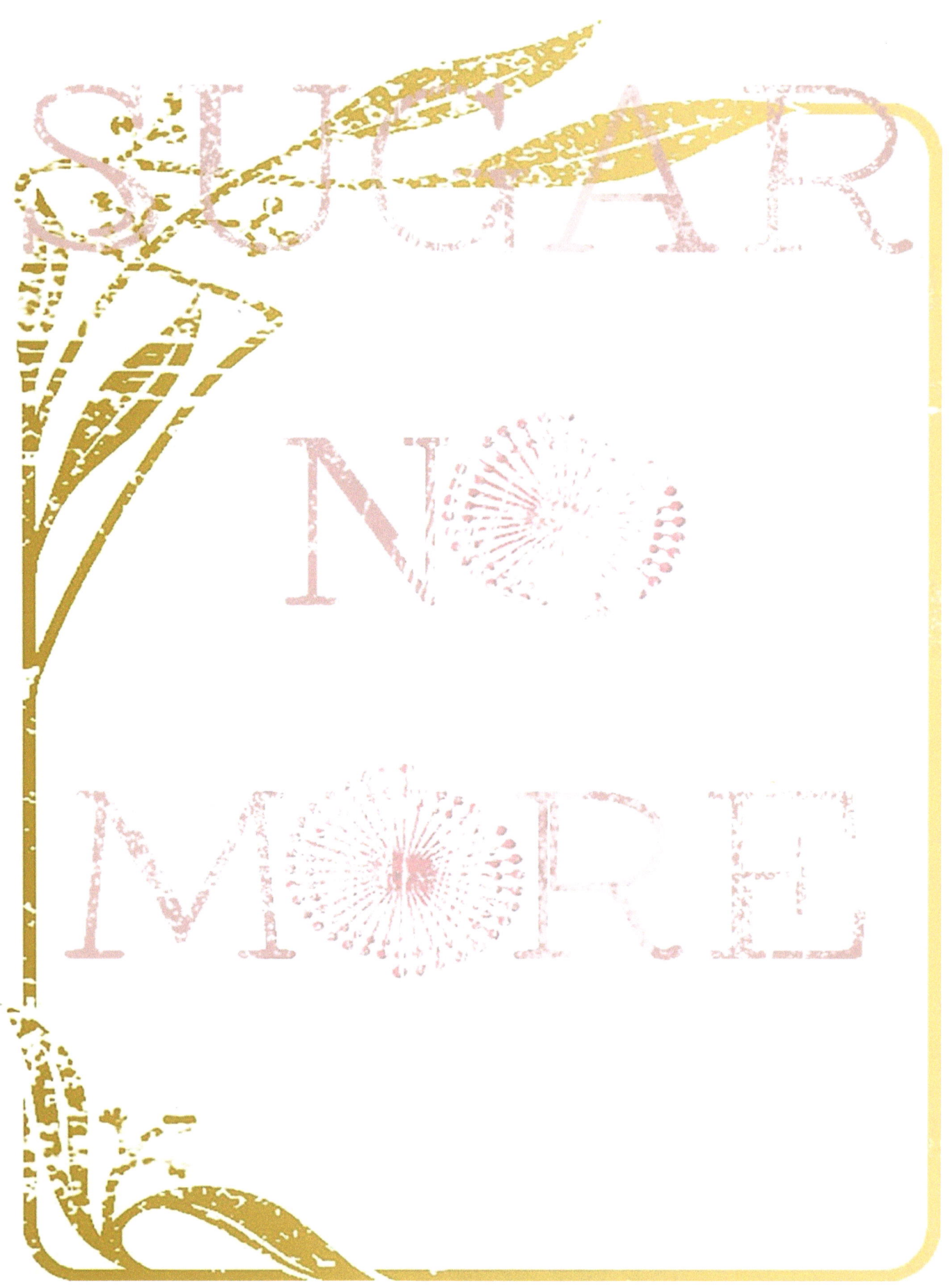

I AM NOT A VICTIM TO SUGAR

About the Author

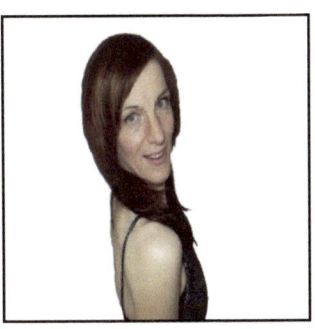

Christine Anderson is an author of integrity with a desire to help others achieve personal and sometimes private health goals, with maximum encouragement and minimum fuss.

For myself, I started eliminating sugar out of my life counseling myself in a firm and definite way, endeavoring to give up sugar primarily for my weight and how I wanted to look. I almost gave up altogether, as it seemed impossible. I knew it could be done, but how? I thought that I had a challenge that I was unable to fully solve, even for a lifetime. I almost gave up in despair and despondency. One day in a flash of inspiration, the idea for this book came forth. From a place of quiet success, knowing that it is possible to coach myself to think and feel differently, about things that are important to me.

The Book

A definite and determined approach was required. I had to have a targeted answer that I could see and to go with it. To do this meant writing it down in big bold letters, to look at as often as possible and allow those words to make me feel constant and strong, able to achieve what I had seen in print, "Sugar no more Lookbook", emerged!

The days that I did not look at the text, were the days that I was eating more sugar. Out came the Lookbook in front of my eyes on its own upright stand, it was beginning to work for me, wow! Yes! I would take this seriously. The written word was purifying my body from sugar.

The Lookbook on the stand in my home is helping me day by day to stop reaching for sugar. This book made it more real and tangible, something that I had not experienced before. I found a solution I liked.

Looking at the answer day by day soothed me, I realised that I could Lookbook my way through the intense times of sugar craving and feel triumphant at small achievements of saying no to a biscuit, or to a spoonful of sugar, quickly and easily. Small steps forward. Sugar no more was working for its place in my daily life.

The Goal

I began to crave not more sugar, but more depth and inner satisfaction of how to bring myself through the demanding times of desiring to take sugar. Finally, seeing it written down, believing it is very much achieving it. I am very happy in my own quest. I have achieved what I set out to do, but I cannot be complacent, hence Lookbook 2 is in the creating and will spring forth into the arena of life, enhancing and liberating.

Victory and Thanks

Christine Anderson ©
ISBN 9780993355042
UK Copyright Service Registered: No 284695148